THE COMPLETE LIVER CIRRHOSIS DIET COOKBOOK 2024

Quick and Easy Friendly Recipes to Improve your Liver and Overall Health

Dr. Raphael Rachelle

TABLE OF CONTENTS

ENCOURAGEMENT

Embracing a liver-friendly lifestyle is not just a commitment to your body; it's a pledge to a life filled with vitality and well-being. As you embark on this journey, remember that every wholesome meal, every nutrient-rich choice is a small victory in the grand narrative of your health.

Picture each plate as a canvas, and your ingredients as the vibrant strokes of a masterpiece, painting a portrait of nourishment and resilience. Your liver is your steadfast ally in this journey, and adopting a liver-friendly lifestyle is akin to offering it the care and attention it deserves.

See every nutrient-packed bite as an investment in your future, a gesture of self-love that ripples through your entire being. Your body, this incredible vessel, thrives on balance and nourishment. By choosing foods that support liver health, you're giving your body the tools it needs to function optimally, to flourish, and to carry you through the adventures of life.

Remember, this is not a restrictive path but a liberating one. It's an exploration of flavors, a discovery of the multitude of delicious options that contribute to your well-being. Allow yourself to revel in the joy of discovering new recipes, experimenting with ingredients, and relishing the culinary journey that unfolds before you.

As you savor each bite, envision the positive impact on your health. Imagine the vibrant energy coursing through your veins, the glow of well-nourished skin, and the resilience that comes with prioritizing your liver's health. Your body is an incredible instrument, and the liver-friendly lifestyle is the harmonious melody that keeps it in tune.

Celebrate your minor successes and try not to be too hard on yourself.

Every step you take towards a liver-friendly lifestyle is a step towards longevity, vitality, and a life well-lived. Embrace this journey with open arms, savor the flavors of well-being, and revel in the incredible transformation that awaits you. Your body will thank you, not just today, but for many vibrant tomorrows to come.

INTRODUCTION

In the bustling heart of a city filled with dreams, Rachael found herself at a crossroads. Battling the challenges of liver cirrhosis, she yearned for a path toward health and vitality. It was in the quiet corners of her kitchen that she discovered the transformative power of **"The Complete Liver Cirrhosis Diet Cookbook 2024."**

As the pages turned, Rachael embarked on a culinary journey that not only tantalized her taste buds but also revitalized her body. With each carefully crafted recipe, she embraced a symphony of flavors that danced on her palate while nurturing her liver back to life. The cookbook became more than just a collection of dishes; it became her compass to success.

Morning rituals of nutrient-rich smoothies and wholesome breakfasts set the tone for her day, fueling her with the energy needed to conquer challenges. Each lunch and dinner became a celebration of fresh, vibrant ingredients carefully chosen to support her liver's healing journey. From mouthwatering grilled salmon to aromatic quinoa bowls, every recipe became a stepping stone toward her triumph over liver cirrhosis.

But this journey wasn't just about recipes; it was a tale of resilience, empowerment, and the sweet taste of victory.

As Rachael navigated through the pages, she discovered the art of cooking for health wasn't just a duty – it was a joy. The kitchen transformed into her sanctuary, and each dish she prepared became a testament to her commitment to well-being.

As the seasons changed, so did Rachael's health. Her perseverance, guided by the wisdom within the cookbook, reflected in medical reports that echoed success. The once-daunting diagnosis became a testament to the incredible potential of a liver-friendly lifestyle. The book, once a guide, became a symbol of triumph over adversity.

In this gastronomic journey, Rachael discovered that the real magic wasn't just in the ingredients but in the transformation she underwent. This was not merely a book—it was the unwavering companion on her road to success, a roadmap to reclaiming her health, and a reminder that every meal could be a step closer to a vibrant, thriving life.

Brief overview of Liver Cirrhosis

Liver cirrhosis is a progressive and irreversible condition characterized by the scarring of the liver tissue, leading to impaired liver function. This disease develops over time, often as a result of chronic liver conditions such as chronic hepatitis, excessive alcohol consumption, or fatty liver disease. As the liver becomes scarred, its ability to perform vital functions, such as detoxification and nutrient processing, is compromised.

The scarring in cirrhosis is the result of long-term liver damage, which can be caused by inflammation and the death of liver cells. This damage triggers a wound-healing response that leads to the formation of fibrous tissue, gradually replacing healthy liver tissue. As cirrhosis progresses, the liver's structure becomes nodular, hindering blood flow and impairing the organ's ability to carry out essential tasks.

Liver cirrhosis is often asymptomatic in its early stages, but as the disease advances, symptoms may include fatigue, weakness, easy bruising, jaundice, and fluid retention. Complications can arise, such as portal hypertension, liver failure, and an increased risk of liver cancer.

Managing liver cirrhosis involves addressing the underlying causes, adopting a liver-friendly diet, and making lifestyle changes. Early detection and intervention play a crucial role in slowing down the progression of cirrhosis and improving the quality of life for individuals affected by this condition.

Importance of Diet in Managing Liver Cirrhosis

Minimizing Liver Strain:

Certain foods can exacerbate liver damage, and a proper diet helps in reducing the burden on the liver. This is particularly important as a compromised liver struggles to process certain substances effectively.

Promoting Nutrient Intake:

A well-balanced diet ensures an adequate intake of essential nutrients, including vitamins, minerals, and proteins. These nutrients are vital for the maintenance and repair of liver cells, contributing to overall liver function.

Managing Complications:

A liver-friendly diet can help manage complications associated with cirrhosis, such as fluid retention (edema) and ascites. Controlling sodium intake, for example, is crucial in reducing fluid accumulation.

Preventing Malnutrition:

Cirrhosis can lead to malnutrition due to a combination of factors, including decreased appetite and nutrient malabsorption. A carefully planned diet helps prevent malnutrition, ensuring the body receives the necessary energy and nutrients.

Addressing Protein Intake:

Protein metabolism can be impaired in individuals with cirrhosis, leading to issues like hepatic encephalopathy.

Managing protein intake is essential to prevent complications while ensuring a sufficient supply of amino acids for overall health.

Controlling Weight:

Maintaining a healthy weight is crucial for individuals with cirrhosis. An appropriate diet can help prevent excessive weight loss or obesity, both of which can contribute to complications associated with liver cirrhosis.

Reducing Inflammation:

Some foods possess anti-inflammatory properties, which can be beneficial for individuals with cirrhosis as inflammation contributes to liver damage. A diet rich in antioxidants and anti-inflammatory foods can help mitigate this risk.

Preventing Fatty Liver:

For individuals with cirrhosis resulting from non-alcoholic fatty liver disease (NAFLD), dietary changes are essential to prevent further fat accumulation in the liver and halt the progression of the disease.

Supporting Overall Health:

A nutritious diet not only supports liver function but also contributes to overall health. This is particularly important for individuals with cirrhosis, as a healthy body is better equipped to cope with the challenges associated with liver disease.

Liver Cirrhosis and Its Causes

Explanation of Liver Cirrhosis:

Liver cirrhosis is a chronic and progressive liver disease characterized by the gradual replacement of healthy liver tissue with scar tissue, leading to impaired liver function. This scarring is the result of long-term damage to the liver, causing inflammation and the death of liver cells. As the liver attempts to repair itself, fibrous tissue forms, disrupting the normal structure of the organ. Over time, this can lead to a nodular and hardened liver, hindering its ability to perform essential functions.

Causes of Liver Cirrhosis:

1. **Chronic Viral Hepatitis:**

   - Hepatitis B and C infections are major contributors to liver cirrhosis. Chronic viral hepatitis causes ongoing inflammation, which can lead to progressive liver damage over time.

2. **Excessive Alcohol Consumption:**

   - Prolonged and excessive alcohol intake is a common cause of cirrhosis. Alcohol-induced liver damage results from the toxic effects of alcohol on liver cells, leading to inflammation, fatty liver, and eventually cirrhosis.

3. **Non-Alcoholic Fatty Liver Disease (NAFLD):**

   - NAFLD is characterized by fat accumulation in the liver and is frequently related with obesity and metabolic syndrome. In its advanced stages, NAFLD can progress to cirrhosis, particularly in individuals with non-alcoholic steatohepatitis (NASH).

4. **Chronic Liver Diseases:**

   - Conditions such as autoimmune hepatitis, primary biliary cirrhosis, and hemochromatosis can contribute to cirrhosis. These diseases involve the immune system mistakenly attacking liver cells or the accumulation of excess iron in the liver.

5. **Genetic Disorders:**

   - Genetic conditions, such as Wilson's disease and cystic fibrosis, can lead to the accumulation of copper or other substances in the liver, causing cirrhosis over time.

6. **Biliary Cirrhosis:**

   - Diseases affecting the bile ducts, such as primary biliary cirrhosis or primary sclerosing cholangitis, can result in cirrhosis by impairing the flow of bile from the liver.

7. **Long-Term Medication Use:**

- Prolonged exposure to certain medications, such as methotrexate or isoniazid, can contribute to liver damage and cirrhosis in some cases.

8. **Vascular Disorders:**

- Conditions affecting blood flow to the liver, such as Budd-Chiari syndrome, can lead to cirrhosis by causing congestion in the liver's blood vessels.

9. **Cystic Fibrosis:**

- This genetic disorder can affect the liver and lead to the development of cirrhosis, particularly in childhood.

Impact of Cirrhosis on the Liver

1. **Structural Changes:**

   - Cirrhosis is characterized by the formation of fibrous scar tissue in the liver, replacing normal, healthy tissue. This scarring disrupts the liver's architecture, leading to a nodular and lumpy appearance. As cirrhosis progresses, the liver becomes harder and more irregular in shape.

2. **Impaired Blood Flow:**

   - The scar tissue in cirrhotic liver acts as a barrier to the normal flow of blood through the organ. This impedes the circulation of blood within the liver, leading to increased pressure in the portal vein—a condition known as portal hypertension. Portal hypertension can result in complications such as varices, ascites, and splenomegaly.

3. **Disruption of Liver Function:**

   - The liver plays a crucial role in numerous physiological functions, including detoxification, metabolism, and the synthesis of proteins. Cirrhosis disrupts these functions, impairing the liver's ability to process toxins, produce essential proteins, and regulate hormones and metabolic pathways.

4. **Altered Detoxification:**

- The liver is a primary organ for detoxifying the body by breaking down and removing toxins. In cirrhosis, the compromised liver struggles to perform this function efficiently, leading to an accumulation of harmful substances in the bloodstream.

5. **Bile Duct Dysfunction:**

- Cirrhosis can cause damage to the bile ducts, which are responsible for transporting bile from the liver to the gallbladder and small intestine. This dysfunction can result in the accumulation of bile in the liver, contributing to further damage.

6. **Risk of Infections:**

- The liver is vital for the immune system, and cirrhosis compromises the organ's ability to fight infections. Individuals with cirrhosis are more susceptible to bacterial infections, which can lead to severe complications.

7. **Fluid Retention:**

- Portal hypertension and liver dysfunction contribute to fluid retention in the abdominal cavity, a condition known as ascites. This accumulation of fluid can lead to abdominal swelling and discomfort.

8. **Risk of Liver Cancer:**

- Cirrhosis is a major risk factor for the development of hepatocellular carcinoma (HCC), a form of liver cancer. The continuous cycle of liver cell death and regeneration in cirrhosis increases the likelihood of malignant transformation.

9. **Cognitive Impairment:**

- In advanced stages, cirrhosis can lead to hepatic encephalopathy, a condition characterized by cognitive dysfunction and neurological symptoms. Elevated levels of toxins, such as ammonia, in the bloodstream contribute to this neurological impairment.

Symptoms and Complications

1. **Fatigue and Weakness:**

   - Individuals with cirrhosis often experience persistent fatigue and weakness due to the compromised ability of the liver to store and release energy.

2. **Jaundice:**

   - Cirrhosis can lead to the buildup of bilirubin in the bloodstream, causing yellowing of the skin and eyes (jaundice).

3. **Fluid Retention:**

   - Portal hypertension can result in the accumulation of fluid in the abdominal cavity, causing swelling and discomfort, a condition known as ascites.

4. **Easy Bruising and Bleeding:**

   - Impaired liver function can lead to a decrease in the production of clotting factors, increasing the risk of easy bruising and bleeding.

5. **Itchy Skin:**

   - The buildup of toxins in the bloodstream can cause itching (pruritus) in individuals with cirrhosis.

6. Loss of Appetite and Weight Loss:

- Cirrhosis can lead to a loss of appetite, nausea, and weight loss due to the impact on nutrient metabolism.

7. Changes in Bowel Habits:

- Cirrhosis can cause changes in bowel movements, including diarrhea or constipation.

8. Confusion and Cognitive Impairment:

- Hepatic encephalopathy, a complication of cirrhosis, can result in confusion, forgetfulness, and difficulty concentrating.

9. Spider Angiomas:

- Small, spider-like blood vessels may become visible on the skin, especially on the upper body.

Complications of Cirrhosis:

1. Portal Hypertension:

- Increased pressure in the portal vein can lead to complications such as varices (enlarged veins in the esophagus or stomach), which are at risk of bleeding.

2. Ascites:

- Fluid accumulation in the abdominal cavity (ascites) can lead to abdominal swelling and discomfort.

3. **Hepatic Encephalopathy:**

- Cognitive dysfunction and neurological symptoms can occur due to the buildup of toxins, particularly ammonia, in the bloodstream.

4. **Hepatorenal Syndrome:**

- Kidney function may be impaired as a result of cirrhosis, leading to hepatorenal syndrome.

5. **Hepatocellular Carcinoma (HCC):**

- Cirrhosis increases the risk of developing liver cancer, particularly hepatocellular carcinoma.

6. **Infections:**

- The compromised immune function in cirrhosis increases the susceptibility to bacterial infections, such as spontaneous bacterial peritonitis.

7. **Bone Disease:**

- Cirrhosis can lead to osteoporosis and other bone disorders due to imbalances in calcium and vitamin D metabolism.

8. **Gastrointestinal Bleeding:**

- Varices associated with portal hypertension can rupture, leading to potentially life-threatening gastrointestinal bleeding.

9. **Malnutrition:**

- Impaired nutrient absorption and metabolism in cirrhosis can result in malnutrition.

10. **Liver Failure:**

- In advanced stages, cirrhosis can progress to liver failure, a life-threatening condition requiring immediate medical attention.

Nutrients Essential for Liver Health

1. **Antioxidants:**

   - **Sources:** Berries, citrus fruits, tomatoes, leafy greens.

   - **Importance:** Antioxidants protect the liver from oxidative stress and inflammation, helping to maintain healthy liver cells.

2. **Omega-3 Fatty Acids:**

   - Fatty fish (salmon, mackerel), flaxseeds, chia seeds, and walnuts are good sources.

   - **Importance:** Omega-3 fatty acids reduce inflammation and may help prevent fatty liver disease.

3. **Vitamin E:**

   - **Sources:** Nuts, seeds, spinach, broccoli.

   - **Importance:** Vitamin E is an antioxidant that helps protect liver cells from damage.

4. **Vitamin C:**

   - **Sources:** Citrus fruits, strawberries, bell peppers.

   - **Importance:** Vitamin C supports the immune system and helps the liver detoxify harmful substances.

5. **B Vitamins:**

- **Sources:** Whole grains, legumes, nuts, seeds, lean meats.

- **Importance:** B vitamins, including B12, B6, and folate, are involved in energy metabolism and help prevent liver damage.

6. **Iron:**

- Lean meat products, lentils, beans, and fortified cereals are all good sources.

- **Importance:** Iron is essential for the formation of hemoglobin and plays a role in preventing anemia, which can be a concern in liver disease.

7. **Zinc:**

- **Sources:** Meat, dairy, nuts, seeds.

- **Importance:** Zinc supports immune function and plays a role in wound healing, important for liver repair.

8. **Selenium:**

- **Sources:** Brazil nuts, fish, turkey, whole grains.

- **Importance:** Selenium is an antioxidant that helps protect the liver from damage.

9. **Magnesium:**

- Leafy greens, nuts, seeds, and whole grains are all good sources.

- **Importance:** Magnesium plays a role in over 300 enzymatic reactions, including those involved in liver function.

10. **Amino Acids (Protein):**

- **Lean meats, fish, eggs, dairy, and legumes are all good sources.**

- **Importance:** Amino acids are building blocks for proteins and support various functions in the liver, including detoxification.

11. **Choline:**

- **Sources:** Eggs, liver, peanuts, soy products.

- **Importance:** Choline is involved in fat metabolism and helps prevent the accumulation of fat in the liver.

12. **Fiber:**

- **Sources:** Whole grains, fruits, vegetables, legumes.

- **Importance:** Dietary fiber aids digestion and helps regulate blood sugar levels, reducing the risk of fatty liver disease.

Key Ingredients for Liver Health

1. **Fatty Fish:**

   - **Examples:** Salmon, mackerel, sardines.

   - **Benefits:** Rich in omega-3 fatty acids, which have anti-inflammatory properties and may help reduce fat accumulation in the liver.

2. **Leafy Greens:**

   - **Examples:** Spinach, kale, collard greens.

   - **Benefits:** High in antioxidants, vitamins (such as vitamin K), and fiber, supporting overall liver function and detoxification.

3. **Cruciferous Vegetables:**

   - **Examples:** Broccoli, cauliflower, Brussels sprouts.

   - **Benefits:** Contain compounds that support detoxification processes in the liver.

4. **Berries:**

   - **Examples:** Blueberries, strawberries, raspberries.

   - **Benefits:** Rich in antioxidants, which help protect liver cells from oxidative stress.

5. **Nuts and Seeds:**

   - **Examples:** Walnuts, flaxseeds, chia seeds.

   - **Benefits:** Provide healthy fats, fiber, and antioxidants that support liver function and reduce inflammation.

6. **Turmeric:**

- **Benefits:** Contains curcumin, which has anti-inflammatory and antioxidant properties, potentially supporting liver health.

7. **Garlic:**

- **Benefits:** Contains allicin, a compound with antioxidant and anti-inflammatory properties that may help protect the liver.

8. **Ginger:**

- **Benefits:** Has anti-inflammatory properties and may contribute to liver protection.

9. **Green Tea:**

- **Benefits:** Contains catechins, antioxidants that may help protect the liver and promote overall health.

10. **Olive Oil:**

- **Benefits:** Provides monounsaturated fats and antioxidants, supporting a healthy liver.

11. **Avocado:**

- **Benefits:** Rich in healthy fats, vitamins, and antioxidants, promoting liver health.

12. **Lean Proteins:**

- **Examples:** Chicken, turkey, tofu.

- **Benefits:** Provide essential amino acids necessary for liver function without excess saturated fats.

13.   **Beets:**

- **Benefits:** Contain betaine, which may help reduce fat buildup in the liver and support liver detoxification.

14.   **Citrus Fruits:**

- **Examples:** Oranges, lemons, grapefruits.

- **Benefits:** High in vitamin C and antioxidants, supporting the immune system and liver health.

15.   **Whole Grains:**

- **Examples:** Quinoa, brown rice, oats.

- **Benefits:** Provide complex carbohydrates, fiber, and B vitamins, supporting overall health and energy metabolism.

16.   **Yogurt and Fermented Foods:**

- **Examples:** Greek yogurt, kefir, sauerkraut.

- **Benefits:** Rich in probiotics that support gut health, which is linked to liver health.

Cooking Techniques for Liver Health

1. Grilling and Broiling:

- **Benefits:** Grilling and broiling cook food quickly and allow excess fats to drip away. This method is suitable for lean proteins like fish and poultry.

2. Steaming:

- **Benefits:** Steaming retains the maximum nutrients in vegetables, fish, and other foods. It requires minimal added fats, making it a liver-friendly cooking technique.

3. Sautéing with Healthy Oils:

- **Benefits:** Use heart-healthy oils like olive oil or avocado oil for sautéing. This method adds flavor without compromising nutritional quality.

4. Baking and Roasting:

- **Benefits:** Baking and roasting help retain nutrients in foods and develop natural flavors. It's a great method for vegetables, whole grains, and lean proteins.

5. Poaching:

- **Benefits:** Poaching involves cooking in simmering liquid, such as water or broth. It's a gentle method suitable for delicate proteins like fish and eggs, preserving their nutritional value.

6. Slow Cooking:

- **Benefits:** Slow cooking at low temperatures allows flavors to meld while keeping the food moist. It's suitable for lean meats, legumes, and hearty vegetables.

7. Stir-Frying:

- **Benefits:** Stir-frying involves quickly cooking small pieces of food in a minimal amount of oil. Use heart-healthy oils and load up on colorful vegetables for added nutrients.

8. Blanching:

- **Benefits:** Blanching involves briefly boiling vegetables and then quickly cooling them. This helps retain color, texture, and nutrients while reducing the overall cooking time.

9. Grating and Chopping:

- **Benefits:** Finely chopping or grating ingredients can reduce cooking time and make nutrients more accessible. This is particularly useful for vegetables that are rich in antioxidants.

10. Using Herbs and Spices:

- **Benefits:** Enhance flavor without relying on excessive salt, sugar, or unhealthy fats. Many herbs and spices have anti-inflammatory properties that can be beneficial for liver health.

11. Minimizing Processed Ingredients:

- **Benefits:** Opt for fresh, whole ingredients rather than processed ones. Processed foods may contain additives and unhealthy fats that can negatively impact liver health.

12. Portion Control:

- **Benefits:** Controlling portion sizes helps prevent overeating, which can contribute to weight management and support overall liver health.

13. Avoiding High-Temperature Cooking with Unhealthy Oils:

- **Benefits:** Limit the use of oils with a low smoke point, such as vegetable oil. High-temperature cooking with unhealthy oils can produce harmful compounds.

14. Incorporating Liver-Friendly Ingredients:

- **Benefits:** Include foods that are known to be beneficial for liver health, such as cruciferous vegetables, garlic, turmeric, and foods high in omega-3 fatty acids.

Food to Include, Limit and Avoid

Foods to Include:

1. **Fruits and Vegetables:**

   - Include a variety of colorful fruits and vegetables for a range of vitamins, minerals, and antioxidants.

2. **Whole Grains:**

   - Opt for whole grains such as brown rice, quinoa, oats, and whole wheat for fiber and essential nutrients.

3. **Lean Proteins:**

   - Choose lean protein sources like poultry, fish, tofu, beans, legumes, and low-fat dairy for muscle maintenance and repair.

4. **Healthy Fats:**

   - Include avocados, nuts, seeds, and olive oil as sources of healthy fats for heart health and nutritional absorption.

5. **Dairy or Dairy Alternatives:**

   - Incorporate low-fat or fat-free dairy products or fortified dairy alternatives for calcium and vitamin D.

6. **Fish:**

   - Include fatty fish like salmon, mackerel, or sardines for omega-3 fatty acids, which are beneficial for heart health.

7. **Nuts and Seeds:**

   - Enjoy moderate amounts of nuts and seeds for healthy fats, protein, and various nutrients.

8. **Water:**

   - Stay hydrated by drinking plenty of water throughout the day for overall health and proper bodily functions.

9. **Herbs and Spices:**

   - Use herbs and spices to flavor meals instead of excessive salt or high-calorie sauces.

10. **Fiber-Rich Foods:**

    - Include fiber-rich foods like beans, lentils, whole grains, fruits, and vegetables to support digestive health.

Foods to Limit:

1. **Processed Foods:**

   - Limit the intake of processed and packaged foods high in added sugars, salt, and unhealthy fats.

2. **Added Sugars:**

- Reduce the consumption of sugary beverages, candies, and processed foods with added sugars.

3. **Saturated Fats:**

- Saturated fats, such as those found in fatty cuts of meat, full-fat dairy and processed foods, should be avoided.

4. **Trans Fats:**

- Avoid trans fats by limiting the intake of partially hydrogenated oils found in some processed and fried foods.

5. **Highly Processed Meats:**

- Limit the intake of processed meats like sausages, hot dogs, and bacon, which may contain preservatives.

6. **Alcohol:**

- Consume alcohol in moderation, if at all, and be mindful of its impact on overall health.

7. **Sodium:**

- Limit the use of table salt and reduce the intake of high-sodium processed foods.

8. **Refined Carbohydrates:**

   - Reduce the consumption of refined carbohydrates like white bread, white rice, and sugary cereals.

9. **High-Caffeine Beverages:**

   - Limit the intake of high-caffeine beverages and consider choosing healthier options like herbal teas.

10. **Artificial Sweeteners:**

    - Use artificial sweeteners in moderation, as some studies suggest potential health concerns with excessive consumption.

Foods to Avoid:

1. **Trans Fats:**

   - Avoid foods containing trans fats, which are linked to an increased risk of heart disease.

2. **Excessive Added Sugars:**

   - Avoid foods and beverages with excessively high added sugar content, which can contribute to various health issues.

3. **Highly Processed and Fried Foods:**

   - Minimize the consumption of highly processed and fried foods that often lack nutritional value.

4. Sugary Beverages:

- Steer clear of sugary sodas, energy drinks, and other high-calorie beverages with little nutritional benefit.

5. Excessive Alcohol:

- Limit alcohol consumption, and avoid binge drinking, which can have adverse health effects.

6. Highly Processed Meats:

- Minimize the intake of highly processed and preserved meats due to potential health risks.

7. Artificial Additives:

- Avoid foods with excessive artificial additives, colors, and preservatives when possible.

8. Unhealthy Cooking Oils:

- Avoid the use of unhealthy cooking oils with a high content of saturated or trans fats.

9. High-Sodium Foods:

- Be cautious of foods high in sodium, especially those from fast-food establishments and certain processed foods.

10. Unhealthy Snacks:

- Limit or avoid unhealthy snacks like chips, candies, and pastries with low nutritional value.

Low-sodium and low-fat alternatives

Low-Sodium Alternatives:

1. **Herbs and Spices:**

   - Use fresh or dried herbs like basil, oregano, thyme, and rosemary to add flavor without sodium.

2. **Citrus Juice:**

   - Lemon or lime juice can enhance the taste of dishes without the need for excessive salt.

3. **Vinegars:**

   - Balsamic vinegar, red wine vinegar, or apple cider vinegar can provide acidity and depth to your meals.

4. **Garlic and Onions:**

   - These aromatic ingredients add robust flavor to dishes, reducing the need for salt.

5. **Low-Sodium Broths:**

   - Opt for reduced-sodium or homemade broths when preparing soups, stews, and sauces.

6. **Homemade Sauces:**

- Create your own sauces using fresh ingredients, herbs, and spices instead of relying on high-sodium store-bought options.

7. **No-Salt-added Canned Goods:**

- Choose canned vegetables, beans, and tomatoes labeled as "no salt added" to control sodium intake.

8. **Fresh Produce:**

- Whole, fresh fruits and vegetables are naturally low in sodium and rich in nutrients.

Low-Fat Alternatives:

1. **Lean Proteins:**

- Choose lean cuts of meat such as chicken or turkey breast, fish, tofu, legumes, and plant-based proteins.

2. **Greek Yogurt:**

- Opt for plain, non-fat Greek yogurt as a substitute for sour cream or mayonnaise in recipes.

3. **Healthy Oils:**

- Use heart-healthy oils like olive oil, avocado oil, or canola oil in moderation.

4. **Avocado:**

- Replace butter or mayonnaise with mashed avocado for a creamy texture and healthy fats.

5. **Low-Fat Dairy:**

- Choose low-fat or fat-free versions of milk, yogurt, and cheese to reduce saturated fat intake.

6. **Whole Grains:**

- For increased fiber and nutrients, use whole grains such as brown rice, quinoa, and whole wheat pasta.

7. **Nuts and Seeds:**

- While high in healthy fats, nuts and seeds can be included in moderation for added nutritional benefits.

8. **Egg Whites:**

- Use egg whites instead of whole eggs to reduce cholesterol and saturated fat content.

9. **Cottage Cheese:**

- Opt for low-fat or fat-free cottage cheese as a protein-rich, lower-fat alternative.

10. **Homemade Dressings:**

- Make your own salad dressings using olive oil, vinegar, and herbs instead of store-bought dressings high in saturated fats.

Managing Specific Dietary Challenge

Reducing Sodium Intake:

- **Strategy:**

    - Choose fresh, whole foods.

    - Use herbs, spices, and citrus for flavor.

    - Read food labels for sodium content.

    - Limit processed and pre-packaged foods.

- **Example:**

- Fresh fruits and vegetables should be used instead of packaged snacks.

2. Lowering Saturated Fat Consumption:

- **Strategy:**

    - Choose lean protein sources.

    - Use healthy oils in moderation.

    - Select low-fat dairy options.

    - Limit red meat and processed meats.

- **Example:**

    - Replace beef burgers with grilled chicken or plant-based alternatives.

3. Managing Diabetes:

- **Strategy:**

  - Focus on portion control.
  - Choose complex carbohydrates.
  - Monitor blood sugar levels regularly.
  - Include fiber-rich foods in meals.

- **Example:**

  - Swap white rice for quinoa or brown rice.

4. Controlling Blood Pressure:

- **Strategy:**

  - Adopt the DASH diet (Dietary Approaches to Stop Hypertension).
  - Reduce sodium intake.
  - Increase potassium-rich foods (fruits, vegetables, beans).
  - Maintain a healthy weight.

- **Example:**

  - Snack on fresh fruit instead of processed snacks.

5. Managing Food Allergies:

- **Strategy:**

  - Read ingredient labels carefully.

- Communicate dietary needs to restaurants.
- Be aware of cross-contamination risks.
- Carry allergy-friendly snacks when needed.

- **Example:**

- Replace peanut butter with sunflower seed butter.

6. Addressing Gluten Sensitivity or Celiac Disease:

- **Strategy:**

- Choose gluten-free grains (quinoa, rice).
- Opt for gluten-free versions of products.
- Be cautious of cross-contamination.
- Focus on naturally gluten-free foods.

- **Example:**

- Substitute regular pasta with gluten-free pasta.

7. Boosting Iron Intake (Iron Deficiency Anemia):

- **Strategy:**

- Consume iron-rich foods (lean meats, beans, spinach).
- Combine iron sources with vitamin C for better absorption.
- Avoid excessive caffeine during meals.
- Consider iron supplements as advised by a healthcare professional.

- **Example:**

  - Pair lentils with bell peppers for increased iron absorption.

8. Weight Management:

- **Strategy:**

  - Focus on balanced, nutrient-dense meals.
  - Practice mindful eating.
  - Incorporate regular physical activity.
  - Set realistic and sustainable goals.

- **Example:**

  - Replace sugary beverages with water or herbal tea.

9. Vegetarian or Vegan Lifestyle:

- **Strategy:**

  - Ensure sufficient protein intake from plant-based sources.
  - Incorporate plenty of fruits and veggies, as well as nuts and seeds
  - Consider fortified foods or supplements for nutrients like B12.
  - Plan meals to cover all essential nutrients.

- **Example:**

  - Make a protein-rich quinoa and black bean salad.

Breakfast options for a liver-friendly starts

Oatmeal with Berries:

Ingredients:

- 1/2 cup steel-cut oats or rolled oats
- 1 cup water or milk alternative (almond milk, soy milk)
- Fresh berries (blueberries, strawberries, raspberries)
- 1 tablespoon chopped nuts (walnuts or almonds)

Instructions:

1. Cook oats according to package instructions using water or your preferred milk.
2. Top with fresh berries and chopped nuts.
3. Stir well and enjoy.

Greek Yogurt Parfait:

Ingredients:

- 1 cup Greek yogurt
- 1/4 cup low-sugar granola
- Sliced banana or berries

- Drizzle of honey

Instructions:

1. In a glass or bowl, layer Greek yogurt with granola.

2. Add sliced banana or berries on top.

3. Drizzle with honey and serve.

Avocado Toast:

Ingredients:

- 1 slice whole-grain bread

- 1/2 ripe avocado, mashed

- Sliced tomatoes

- Sprinkle of chia seeds

Instructions:

1. Toast the whole-grain bread.

2. Spread mashed avocado on the toast.

3. Top with sliced tomatoes and a sprinkle of chia seeds.

Smoothie Bowl:

Ingredients:

- Handful of spinach or kale

- 1/2 cup frozen berries

- 1 banana
- 1/2 cup Greek yogurt
- 1 tablespoon chia seeds

Instructions:

1. Blend spinach, berries, banana, and Greek yogurt until smooth.
2. Pour into a bowl and sprinkle with chia seeds.
3. Add additional toppings if desired, and enjoy with a spoon.

Egg and Vegetable Omelette:

Ingredients:

- 2 eggs
- Handful of spinach, tomatoes, and bell peppers (or your choice of vegetables)
- 1 tablespoon olive oil
- Herbs and spices for flavor

Instructions

1. In a bowl, whisk eggs and season with herbs and spices.
2. Heat olive oil in a pan, add vegetables, and sauté until tender.
3. Pour whisked eggs over the vegetables, cook until set, then fold in half.

Quinoa Breakfast Bowl:

Ingredients:

- 1/2 cup cooked quinoa
- Sliced banana
- 1 tablespoon chopped nuts (almonds or walnuts)
- Drizzle of honey or maple syrup

Instructions:

1. Cook quinoa according to package instructions.
2. In a bowl, layer cooked quinoa with sliced banana.
3. Sprinkle with chopped nuts and drizzle with honey or maple syrup.

Chia Seed Pudding:

Ingredients:

- 2 tablespoons chia seeds
- 1/2 cup milk or a milk alternative (almond milk, coconut milk)
- Fresh fruit (kiwi, berries)
- Sliced almonds

Instructions:

1. Mix chia seeds with milk in a bowl and let it sit in the refrigerator for a few hours or overnight until it thickens.

2. Layer chia pudding with fresh fruit in a serving glass.

3. Top with sliced almonds before serving.

Whole Grain Pancakes:

Ingredients:

- Whole-grain pancake mix
- Sliced bananas or berries
- Greek yogurt topping
- Drizzle of honey

Instructions:

1. Prepare pancakes according to the whole-grain pancake mix instructions.
2. Top pancakes with sliced bananas or berries.

3. Drizzle with honey and top with a dollop of Greek yogurt.

Salmon and Cream Cheese Bagel:

Ingredients:

- 1 whole-grain bagel, sliced and toasted
- Smoked salmon
- Cream cheese
- Sliced cucumber and tomato

Instructions:

1. Toast the whole-grain bagel slices.

2. Spread cream cheese on the bagel halves.

3. Layer with smoked salmon, sliced cucumber, and tomato.

Vegetarian Breakfast Burrito:

Ingredients:

- Scrambled eggs or tofu

- Black beans, drained and rinsed

- Salsa

- Avocado slices

- Whole-grain tortilla

Instructions:

1. Cook scrambled eggs or tofu in a pan.

2. Warm the whole-grain tortilla.

3. Assemble the burrito with eggs or tofu, black beans, salsa, and avocado slices. Roll it up and enjoy.

Delicious and Nutrient-Rich Lunch Recipes

Grilled Chicken Salad:

Ingredients:

- Grilled chicken breast, sliced
- Mixed salad greens (spinach, arugula, lettuce)
- Cherry tomatoes, halved
- Cucumber, sliced
- Avocado, diced
- Balsamic vinaigrette dressing

Instructions:

1. Combine grilled chicken, salad greens, tomatoes, cucumber, and avocado in a bowl.

2. Drizzle with balsamic vinaigrette dressing and toss gently.

Quinoa and Vegetable Stir-Fry:

Ingredients:

- Cooked quinoa

- Broccoli florets

- Bell peppers, sliced

- Carrots, julienned

- Edamame beans

- Soy sauce and sesame oil for stir-frying

Instructions:

1. Stir-fry broccoli, bell peppers, carrots, and edamame in a pan with soy sauce and sesame oil.

2. Mix in cooked quinoa and stir until well combined.

Lentil and Vegetable Soup:

Ingredients:

- Red lentils

- Carrots, diced

- Celery, chopped

- Onion, finely chopped

- Vegetable broth

- Herbs and spices (cumin, turmeric, thyme)

- Spinach leaves

Instructions:

1. Cook lentils, carrots, celery, and onion in vegetable broth with herbs and spices.

2. Add spinach leaves just before serving.

Salmon and Quinoa Bowl:

Ingredients:

- Grilled or baked salmon fillet
- Quinoa, cooked
- Steamed broccoli
- Sliced radishes
- Lemon-tahini dressing

Instructions:

1. Assemble a bowl with quinoa, steamed broccoli, and grilled salmon.

2. Top with sliced radishes and drizzle with lemon-tahini dressing.

Chickpea and Spinach Wrap:

Ingredients:

- Whole-grain wrap
- Chickpeas, cooked

- Spinach leaves

- Cherry tomatoes, halved

- Feta cheese, crumbled

- Greek yogurt dressing

Instructions:

1. Fill a whole-grain wrap with chickpeas, spinach, cherry tomatoes, and feta cheese.

2. Drizzle with Greek yogurt dressing and roll up the wrap.

Sweet Potato and Black Bean Bowl:

Ingredients:

- Roasted sweet potato cubes

- Black beans, cooked

- Quinoa, cooked

- Sliced avocado

- Lime-cilantro dressing

Instructions:

1. Combine roasted sweet potato, black beans, and quinoa in a bowl.

2. Top with sliced avocado and drizzle with lime-cilantro dressing.

Turkey and Vegetable Stir-Fry:

Ingredients:

- Lean ground turkey
- Mixed stir-fry vegetables (bell peppers, snap peas, carrots)
- Brown rice, cooked
- Low-sodium soy sauce
- Ginger and garlic for flavor

Instructions:

1. Cook ground turkey in a pan with ginger and garlic.
2. Add stir-fry vegetables and soy sauce, stir until cooked.
3. Serve over cooked brown rice.

Mediterranean Chickpea Salad:

Ingredients:

- Canned chickpeas, drained
- Cherry tomatoes, halved
- Cucumber, diced
- Kalamata olives, sliced
- Feta cheese, crumbled
- Olive oil and lemon dressing

Instructions:

1. Combine chickpeas, tomatoes, cucumber, olives, and feta in a bowl.

2. Drizzle with olive oil and lemon dressing, toss gently.

Shrimp and Quinoa Stuffed Bell Peppers:

Ingredients:

- Bell peppers, halved
- Shrimp, cooked and chopped
- Quinoa, cooked
- Spinach, chopped
- Tomato sauce
- Mozzarella cheese, shredded

Instructions:

1. Precook bell peppers until slightly tender.

2. In a bowl, mix shrimp, quinoa, spinach, and tomato sauce.

3. Stuff bell peppers with the mixture, top with mozzarella, and bake until cheese is melted.

Tofu and Vegetable Noodle Bowl:

Ingredients:

- Rice noodles, cooked
- Firm tofu, cubed and stir-fried
- Broccoli florets
- Carrots, julienned
- Snow peas
- Sesame-ginger dressing

Instructions:

1. Cook rice noodles according to package instructions.

2. Stir-fry tofu, broccoli, carrots, and snow peas in sesame-ginger dressing.

3. Toss with cooked rice noodles before serving.

Nutrient-Rich Dinner Recipes

Baked Lemon Herb Salmon:

Ingredients:

- Salmon fillets
- Lemon juice
- Fresh herbs (such as dill, parsley)
- Olive oil
- Garlic, minced
- Salt and pepper

Instructions:

1. Preheat the oven. Arrange the salmon fillets on a baking sheet

2. Drizzle with olive oil and lemon juice. Season with minced garlic, fresh herbs, salt, and pepper to taste.

3. Bake the salmon till it is cooked thoroughly and flakes readily with a fork.

Quinoa and Black Bean Stuffed Bell Peppers:

Ingredients:

- Bell peppers, halved
- Quinoa, cooked
- Black beans, cooked
- Corn kernels
- Diced tomatoes
- Mexican seasoning
- Shredded cheese

Instructions:

1. Precook bell peppers until slightly tender.

2. In a bowl, mix quinoa, black beans, corn, diced tomatoes, and Mexican seasoning.

3. Stuff bell peppers with the mixture, top with shredded cheese, and bake until cheese is melted.

Veggie Stir-Fry with Tofu:

Ingredients:

- Tofu, cubed
- Mixed stir-fry vegetables (bell peppers, broccoli, snap peas)
- Soy sauce
- Ginger and garlic, minced
- Sesame oil
- Brown rice, cooked

Instructions:

1. Stir-fry tofu, vegetables, ginger, and garlic in sesame oil and soy sauce.

2. Serve over cooked brown rice.

Lentil and Vegetable Curry:

Ingredients:

- Red lentils
- Mixed vegetables (carrots, cauliflower, peas)
- Coconut milk
- Curry spices (turmeric, cumin, coriander)
- Garlic and ginger, minced
- Basmati rice, cooked

Instructions:

1. Cook lentils and vegetables in coconut milk with curry spices, garlic, and ginger.

2. Serve over cooked basmati rice.

Chicken and Quinoa Skillet:

Ingredients:

- Chicken breast, sliced
- Quinoa, cooked
- Spinach leaves
- Cherry tomatoes, halved
- Feta cheese, crumbled
- Olive oil
- Lemon juice

Instructions:

1. Sauté chicken slices in olive oil until cooked.

2. Combine cooked quinoa, spinach, cherry tomatoes, and feta.

3. Top with cooked chicken and drizzle with lemon juice.

Spinach and Mushroom Stuffed Chicken Breast:

Ingredients:

- Chicken breasts
- Fresh spinach
- Mushrooms, sliced
- Garlic, minced
- Feta or goat cheese
- Olive oil
- Salt and pepper

Instructions:

1. Preheat the oven. Butterfly chicken breasts.

2. Sauté mushrooms and garlic in olive oil. Add spinach and cook until wilted.

3. Stuff chicken breasts with the spinach-mushroom mixture

and cheese. Bake until chicken is cooked through.

Sweet Potato and Chickpea Curry:

Ingredients:

- Sweet potatoes, diced
- Chickpeas, cooked
- Coconut milk
- Curry powder
- Onion, diced
- Garlic and ginger, minced
- Cilantro for garnish

Instructions:

1. Cook sweet potatoes, chickpeas, onion, garlic, and ginger in coconut milk with curry powder.

2. Garnish with cilantro before serving.

Mediterranean Quinoa Salad:

Ingredients:

- Quinoa, cooked
- Cherry tomatoes, halved
- Cucumber, diced
- Kalamata olives, sliced
- Feta cheese, crumbled
- Red onion, finely chopped
- Drizzle with a dressing of olive oil and balsamic vinegar.

Instructions:

1. Combine cooked quinoa, tomatoes, cucumber, olives, feta, and red onion.

2. Drizzle with olive oil and balsamic vinegar dressing.

Turkey and Vegetable Skewers:

Ingredients:

- Ground turkey
- Bell peppers, cut into chunks
- Cherry tomatoes
- Red onion, cut into wedges
- Olive oil
- Italian herbs and spices

Instructions:

1. Mix ground turkey with Italian herbs and spices. Form into skewers.

2. Thread turkey skewers with bell peppers, cherry tomatoes, and red onion.

3. Grill or bake until turkey is cooked.

Blackened Shrimp and Quinoa Salad:

Ingredients:

- Blackened shrimp
- Quinoa, cooked
- Avocado, diced
- Cherry tomatoes, halved
- Corn kernels
- Cilantro, chopped
- Lime vinaigrette dressing

Instructions:

1. Toss cooked quinoa with diced avocado, cherry tomatoes, corn, and cilantro.

2. Top with blackened shrimp and drizzle with lime vinaigrette dressing.

Healthy Snacks Recipes

Greek Yogurt Parfait:

Ingredients:

- Greek yogurt
- Mixed berries (blueberries, strawberries)
- Granola
- Honey

Instructions:

1. In a glass or bowl, layer Greek yogurt with mixed berries.

2. Add a sprinkle of granola and drizzle with honey.

Hummus and Veggie Sticks:

Ingredients:

- Hummus
- Carrot sticks
- Cucumber slices
- Cherry tomatoes

Instructions:

1. Dip carrot sticks, cucumber slices, and cherry tomatoes into hummus.

2. Enjoy this crunchy and satisfying snack.

Almond Butter Banana Bites:

Ingredients:

- Banana, sliced
- Almond butter
- Chia seeds

Instructions:

1. Spread almond butter on banana slices.

2. Sprinkle with chia seeds for added crunch and nutrition.

Avocado Toast with Radishes:

Ingredients:

- Whole-grain bread
- Avocado, mashed
- Radishes, thinly sliced
- Sea salt

Instructions:

1. Toast whole-grain bread and spread mashed avocado.

2. Top with thinly sliced radishes and a sprinkle of sea salt.

Trail Mix:

Ingredients:

- Nuts (almonds, walnuts, cashews)
- Seeds (pumpkin seeds, sunflower seeds)
- Dried fruits (raisins, cranberries)
- Dark chocolate chips

Instructions:

1. Mix nuts, seeds, dried fruits, and dark chocolate chips in a bowl.

2. Create individual portions for a convenient and nutritious snack.

Cottage Cheese with Pineapple:

Ingredients:

- Cottage cheese
- Fresh pineapple chunks
- Almonds, chopped

Instructions:

1. Combine cottage cheese with fresh pineapple chunks.

2. To add flavor, toss chopped almonds over the top.

Roasted Chickpeas:

Ingredients:

- Canned chickpeas, drained and rinsed
- Olive oil
- Paprika
- Garlic powder

Instructions:

1. Toss chickpeas in olive oil, paprika, and garlic powder until well coated.
2. Roast in the oven until crispy for a crunchy and protein-packed snack.

Whole Grain Crackers with Tuna Salad:

Ingredients:

- Whole-grain crackers
- Canned tuna, drained
- Greek yogurt
- Dill, chopped
- Lemon juice

Instructions:

1. Mix canned tuna with Greek yogurt, chopped dill, and lemon juice.
2. Serve on top of whole-grain crackers.

Apple Slices with Nut Butter:

Ingredients:

- Apple, sliced
- Almond butter or peanut butter
- Cinnamon

Instructions:

1. Spread almond butter on apple slices.

2. Sprinkle with cinnamon for a tasty and satisfying snack.

Vegetable Roll-Ups:

Ingredients:

- Sliced turkey or chicken
- Hummus
- Bell pepper strips
- Spinach leaves

Instructions:

1. Spread hummus on sliced turkey or chicken.

2. Add bell pepper strips and spinach leaves, then roll up for a protein-packed snack.

Nutrient-Rich desserts Recipes

Berry and Yogurt Parfait:

Ingredients:

- Greek yogurt
- Mixed berries (strawberries, blueberries, raspberries)
- Honey
- Granola

Instructions:

1. In a glass or bowl, layer Greek yogurt with mixed berries.

2. Drizzle with honey and sprinkle with granola.

Dark Chocolate-Dipped Strawberries:

Ingredients:

- Fresh strawberries
- Dark chocolate, melted
- Chopped nuts (almonds, pistachios)

Instructions:

1. Dip each strawberry in melted dark chocolate.

2. Sprinkle with chopped nuts and let them cool until the chocolate hardens.

Chia Seed Pudding with Mango:

Ingredients:

- Chia seeds
- Almond milk
- Mango, diced
- Vanilla extract

Instructions:

1. Chia seeds, almond milk, and vanilla extract should be combined.

2. Refrigerate until it thickens, then layer with diced mango.

Baked Apples with Cinnamon:

Ingredients:

- Apples, cored and sliced
- Cinnamon
- Walnuts, chopped
- Greek yogurt (optional)

Instructions:

1. Arrange apple slices in a baking dish.

2. Sprinkle with cinnamon and chopped walnuts. Bake until tender.

3. If preferred, top with a dollop of Greek yogurt.

Frozen Banana Bites:

Ingredients:

- Bananas, sliced
- Peanut butter
- Dark chocolate, melted
- Coconut flakes

Instructions:

1. Spread peanut butter on banana slices and create sandwiches.

2. Dip each sandwich in melted dark chocolate and sprinkle with coconut flakes.

3. Freeze until firm.

Almond Flour Blueberry Muffins:

Ingredients:

- Almond flour
- Eggs
- Maple syrup
- Baking powder

- Blueberries

Instructions:

1. Mix almond flour, eggs, maple syrup, and baking powder.

2. Fold in blueberries and bake in muffin cups until golden.

Avocado Chocolate Mousse:

Ingredients:

- Avocado
- Cocoa powder
- Maple syrup or honey
- Vanilla extract
- Almond milk

Instructions:

1. Blend avocado, cocoa powder, maple syrup, vanilla extract, and almond milk until smooth.

2. Chill before serving.

Oatmeal Banana Cookies:

Ingredients:

- Ripe bananas, mashed
- Rolled oats
- Raisins or dark chocolate chips
- Cinnamon

Instructions:

1. Mix mashed bananas with rolled oats, raisins or chocolate chips, and cinnamon.

2. Drop spoonfuls onto a baking sheet and bake until golden.

Coconut Chia Pudding:

Ingredients:

- Chia seeds
- Coconut milk
- Maple syrup
- Shredded coconut

Instructions:

1. Combine chia seeds, coconut milk, and maple syrup. Refrigerate until set.

2. Top with shredded coconut before serving.

Pistachio and Cranberry Energy Bites:

Ingredients:

- Dates, pitted
- Pistachios, shelled
- Dried cranberries
- Vanilla extract
- Rolled oats

Instructions:

1. Blend dates, pistachios, cranberries, vanilla extract, and rolled oats in a food processor.

2. Roll the mixture into small energy bites.

Vegetarian Recipes That Cover a Range of Cuisines and Flavors

Vegetarian Chickpea Curry:

Ingredients:

- Chickpeas, cooked
- Tomatoes, diced
- Onion, chopped
- Garlic and ginger, minced
- Coconut milk
- Curry spices (turmeric, cumin, coriander)
- Spinach leaves

Instructions:

1. Sauté onions, garlic, and ginger until fragrant.
2. Add chickpeas, diced tomatoes, coconut milk, and curry spices.
3. Simmer until flavors meld, then stir in fresh spinach before serving.

Caprese Salad Stuffed Avocados:

Ingredients:

- Avocados, halved
- Cherry tomatoes, halved
- Fresh mozzarella, diced
- Fresh basil leaves
- Balsamic glaze
- Salt and pepper

Instructions:

1. To make a well, scoop out some avocado.
2. Mix cherry tomatoes, mozzarella, and basil. Fill avocado halves.
3. Garnish with salt and pepper as well as with balsamic glaze.

Vegetarian Tacos:

Ingredients:

- Black beans, cooked
- Corn tortillas
- Avocado, sliced
- Salsa
- Shredded lettuce
- Cheese

- Lime wedges

Instructions:

1. Warm corn tortillas and fill with black beans, avocado, salsa, lettuce, and cheese.
2. Serve with lime wedges.

Mushroom and Spinach Risotto:

Ingredients:

- Arborio rice
- Mushrooms, sliced
- Spinach leaves
- Vegetable broth
- Parmesan cheese
- White wine
- Onion and garlic, chopped

Instructions:

1. Sauté onions and garlic, then add mushrooms and spinach.
2. Stir in Arborio rice, white wine, and vegetable broth until creamy.
3. Finish with Parmesan cheese.

Quinoa and Black Bean Stuffed Peppers:

Ingredients:

- Bell peppers, halved
- Quinoa, cooked
- Black beans, cooked
- Corn kernels
- Salsa
- Cumin and chili powder
- Shredded cheese

Instructions:

1. Precook bell peppers until slightly tender.
2. Mix quinoa, black beans, corn, salsa, cumin, and chili powder.
3. Stuff peppers and top with shredded cheese. Bake until cheese melts.

Vegetarian Pad Thai:

Ingredients:

- Rice noodles
- Tofu, cubed
- Bean sprouts
- Peanuts, crushed
- Green onions, sliced

- Lime wedges
- Pad Thai sauce

Instructions:

1. Cook rice noodles and set aside.

2. Sauté tofu, add cooked noodles, bean sprouts, and pad Thai sauce.

3. Serve with crushed peanuts, sliced green onions, and lime wedges.

Eggplant Parmesan:

Ingredients:

- Eggplant, sliced
- Marinara sauce
- Mozzarella and Parmesan cheese
- Bread crumbs
- Eggs
- Fresh basil

Instructions:

1. Dip eggplant slices in beaten eggs, coat with bread crumbs, and bake until golden.

2. Layer eggplant with marinara sauce and cheeses. Bake until bubbly.

3. Garnish with fresh basil.

Vegetarian Buddha Bowl:

Ingredients:

- Quinoa, cooked
- Roasted sweet potatoes
- Avocado, sliced
- Chickpeas, roasted
- Shredded cabbage
- Tahini dressing

Instructions:

1. Arrange quinoa, sweet potatoes, avocado, chickpeas, and shredded cabbage in a bowl.
2. Drizzle with tahini dressing.

Cauliflower and Chickpea Curry:

Ingredients:

- Cauliflower florets
- Chickpeas, cooked
- Coconut milk
- Curry spices (turmeric, cumin, garam masala)
- Tomatoes, diced
- Fresh cilantro

Instructions:

- Sauté cauliflower, chickpeas, and spices until tender.

- Add diced tomatoes and coconut milk. Simmer until flavors meld.

- Garnish with fresh cilantro before serving.

Vegetarian Lentil Soup:

Ingredients:

- Lentils, rinsed

- Carrots, diced

- Celery, chopped

- Onion, finely chopped

- Vegetable broth

- Garlic and thyme

- Spinach leaves

Instructions:

1. Cook until the onions, garlic, carrots, and celery are softened.

2. Add lentils, vegetable broth, and thyme. Simmer until lentils are tender.

3. Stir in fresh spinach before serving.

Smoothie Recipes

Green Tropical Smoothie:

Ingredients:

- 1 cup spinach (fresh or frozen)
- 1/2 cup pineapple chunks
- 1/2 banana
- 1/2 cup mango chunks
- 1 cup coconut water
- Ice cubes

Instructions:

1. Blend spinach and coconut water until smooth.
2. Add pineapple, banana, mango, and ice cubes.
3. Blend until creamy and enjoy.

Berry Blast Smoothie:

Ingredients:

- 1 cup mixed berries (strawberries, blueberries, raspberries)
- 1/2 cup Greek yogurt
- 1/2 banana
- 1 tablespoon chia seeds
- 1 cup almond milk
- Ice cubes

Instructions:

1. Combine mixed berries, Greek yogurt, banana, chia seeds, and almond milk in a blender.
2. Blend until smooth, add ice cubes, and blend again.

Mango Ginger Smoothie:

Ingredients:

- 1 cup mango chunks
- 1/2 cup plain yogurt
- 1 teaspoon fresh ginger, grated
- 1 tablespoon honey
- 1 cup coconut water
- Ice cubes

Instructions:

1. Blend mango, yogurt, ginger, honey, and coconut water until smooth.
2. Add ice cubes and blend again.

Peanut Butter Banana Protein Smoothie:

Ingredients:

- 1 banana
- 2 tablespoons peanut butter
- 1 scoop vanilla protein powder
- 1 cup almond milk
- Ice cubes

Instructions:

1. Blend banana, peanut butter, protein powder, and almond milk until well combined.
2. Add ice cubes and blend until smooth.

Citrus Sunshine Smoothie:

Ingredients:

- 1 orange, peeled
- 1/2 cup pineapple chunks
- 1/2 cup Greek yogurt
- 1 tablespoon flaxseeds
- 1 cup water
- Ice cubes

Instructions:

1. Blend orange, pineapple, Greek yogurt, flaxseeds, and water until smooth.
2. Add ice cubes and blend again.

Chocolate Avocado Power Smoothie:

Ingredients:

- 1/2 avocado
- 1 tablespoon cocoa powder
- 1 tablespoon honey
- 1/2 cup spinach
- 1 cup almond milk
- Ice cubes

Instructions:

1. Blend avocado, cocoa powder, honey, spinach, and almond milk until creamy.
2. Add ice cubes and blend until smooth.

Cucumber Mint Cooler Smoothie:

Ingredients:

- 1/2 cucumber, peeled
- 1/2 cup mint leaves
- 1/2 lime, juiced
- 1 cup coconut water
- 1 tablespoon honey
- Ice cubes

Instructions:

1. Blend cucumber, mint leaves, lime juice, coconut water, and honey until well combined.
2. Add ice cubes and blend again.

Blueberry Almond Butter Bliss:

Ingredients:

- 1 cup blueberries (fresh or frozen)
- 2 tablespoons almond butter
- 1/2 banana
- 1 cup almond milk
- Ice cubes

Instructions:

1. Blend blueberries, almond butter, banana, and almond milk until smooth.

2. Add ice cubes and blend until creamy.

Tropical Paradise Smoothie:

Ingredients:

- 1/2 cup mango chunks
- 1/2 cup pineapple chunks
- 1/2 banana
- 1/2 cup coconut milk
- 1/2 cup orange juice
- Ice cubes

Instructions:

1. Blend mango, pineapple, banana, coconut milk, and orange juice until well blended.
2. Add ice cubes and blend until smooth.

Strawberry Kiwi Refresher Smoothie:

Ingredients:

- 1 cup strawberries, hulled
- 2 kiwis, peeled and sliced
- 1/2 cup Greek yogurt
- 1 tablespoon honey
- 1 cup water
- Ice cubes

Instructions

1. Blend strawberries, kiwi, Greek yogurt, honey, and water until smooth.

2. Add ice cubes and blend until refreshing.

BONUS

30 Days of Delicious Healthy Meal Plan

Day	Breakfast	Lunch	Dinner
1	Greek yogurt with berries and granola	Grilled chicken salad with balsamic vinaigrette	Baked salmon with quinoa and steamed broccoli
2	Spinach and feta omelet with whole-grain toast	Lentil soup with mixed green salad	Stir-fried tofu with vegetables and brown rice
3	Overnight oats with almond milk and fruit	Turkey and avocado wrap with whole-grain tortilla	Grilled shrimp with sweet potato wedges and asparagus
4	Peanut Butter Banana Protein Smoothie	Quinoa salad with chickpeas, cucumbers, and tomatoes	Baked chicken with roasted Brussels sprouts and quinoa
5	Whole-grain pancakes with fresh	Caprese salad with mozzarella,	Eggplant and chickpea curry with

Day	Breakfast	Lunch	Dinner
	berries	tomatoes, and basil	brown rice
6	Avocado toast with poached eggs	Spinach and mushroom whole-grain wrap with hummus	Grilled steak with sweet potato mash and green beans
7	Cottage cheese with pineapple chunks	Quinoa-stuffed bell peppers with mixed greens	Baked cod with quinoa pilaf and roasted asparagus
8	Green Tropical Smoothie	Chickpea and vegetable stir-fry with quinoa	Baked tilapia with lemon-dill sauce, sweet potato, and green beans
9	Scrambled eggs with spinach and toast	Turkey and vegetable kebabs with tabbouleh	Lentil and vegetable curry with brown rice
10	Smoothie bowl with berries and granola	Quinoa and black bean bowl with avocado and salsa	Grilled chicken breast with quinoa and roasted Brussels sprouts

Day	Breakfast	Lunch	Dinner
11	Banana and almond butter smoothie	Spinach and feta stuffed chicken breast with a side	Spaghetti squash with marinara sauce and turkey meatballs
12	Oatmeal with sliced strawberries	Shrimp and vegetable stir-fried rice	Baked cod with mango salsa, quinoa, and steamed broccoli
13	Avocado and tomato on whole-grain toast	Greek salad with grilled chicken and pita	Eggplant lasagna with a side of mixed greens
14	Greek yogurt parfait with granola	Black bean and vegetable wrap with cucumber salad	Beef and vegetable stir-fry with brown rice
15	Acai bowl with mixed berries and granola	Turkey and quinoa stuffed bell peppers	Baked salmon with lemon herb sauce, quinoa, and Brussels sprouts
16	Whole-grain bagel with smoked salmon	Lentil and vegetable soup with mixed green salad	Grilled chicken Caesar salad with whole-grain croutons

Day	Breakfast	Lunch	Dinner
17	Smoothie with kale, pineapple, and coconut water	Turkey and avocado salad with honey-mustard dressing	Spaghetti with zucchini noodles and turkey Bolognese sauce
18	Cottage cheese and pineapple smoothie	Caprese quinoa bowl with balsamic glaze	Teriyaki tofu stir-fry with brown rice and broccoli
19	Whole-grain pancakes with sliced strawberries	Chickpea and vegetable curry with basmati rice	Baked cod with mango avocado salsa, quinoa, and steamed asparagus
20	Greek yogurt with mixed berries and nuts	Turkey and cranberry wrap with whole-grain tortilla	Eggplant and chickpea stew with a side of couscous
21	Scrambled eggs with sautéed spinach	Quinoa salad with black beans, corn, avocado, and lime-cilantro dressing	Grilled chicken with sweet potato wedges and green beans
22	Smoothie bowl with	Quinoa and	Grilled shrimp and

Day	Breakfast	Lunch	Dinner
	banana, berries, almond butter, and granola	vegetable sushi rolls with soy sauce	vegetable kebabs with quinoa
23	Whole-grain bagel with smoked salmon, cream cheese, and cucumber slices	Lentil and sweet potato curry with brown rice	Baked chicken breast with rosemary, roasted sweet potatoes, and green beans
24	Smoothie with kale, pineapple, banana, and coconut water	Turkey and avocado salad with honey-mustard dressing	Spaghetti squash primavera with tomato and basil sauce
25	Chia seed pudding with almond milk and kiwi	Caprese-stuffed chicken breast with balsamic glaze and quinoa	Stir-fried tofu with broccoli, bell peppers, and brown rice
26	Whole-grain toast with smashed avocado and poached	Quinoa and black bean stuffed sweet potatoes with salsa	Baked cod with lemon-caper sauce, quinoa, and roasted

Day	Breakfast	Lunch	Dinner
	eggs		Brussels sprouts
27	Greek yogurt parfait with granola, mixed berries, and honey	Chickpea and vegetable stir-fry with brown rice	Grilled steak with chimichurri sauce, sweet potato mash, and asparagus
28	Oatmeal with sliced peaches, almonds, and cinnamon	Spinach and feta stuffed portobello mushrooms with a side salad	Eggplant lasagna rolls with a side of mixed vegetables
29	Smoothie bowl with banana, berries, almond butter, and granola	Quinoa and black bean salad with corn, avocado, and lime-cilantro dressing	Grilled chicken with mango salsa, quinoa, and steamed broccoli
30	Avocado and tomato on whole-grain toast with a poached egg	Spinach and feta stuffed chicken breast with quinoa	Baked salmon with lemon-dill sauce, sweet potato, and green beans

Feel free to customize the plan according to your taste preferences and dietary requirements. This tabular format allows you to easily organize and follow the 30-day meal plan.

www.ingramcontent.com/pod-product-compliance
Lightning Source LLC
Chambersburg PA
CBHW080937260726
48661CB00010B/3959